JUICING

FOR

COLITIS

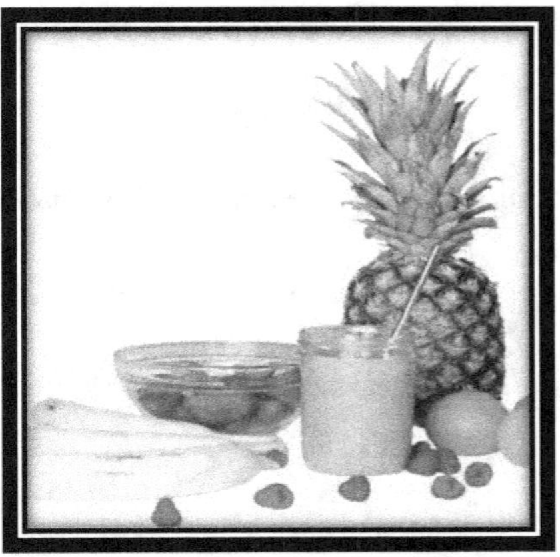

40 Essential and Easy-To-Make Nutrient-Rich Juice Blends for Crohn's, IBD, And Ulcerative Colitis Disease Management

DR. LINDA B. ALLEN

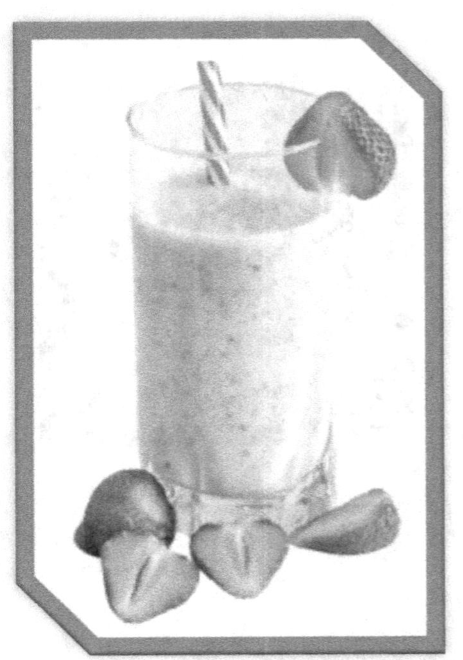

SCAN THE QR-CODE BELOW FOR MORE BOOKS FROM THIS AUTHOR

TABLE OF CONTENTS

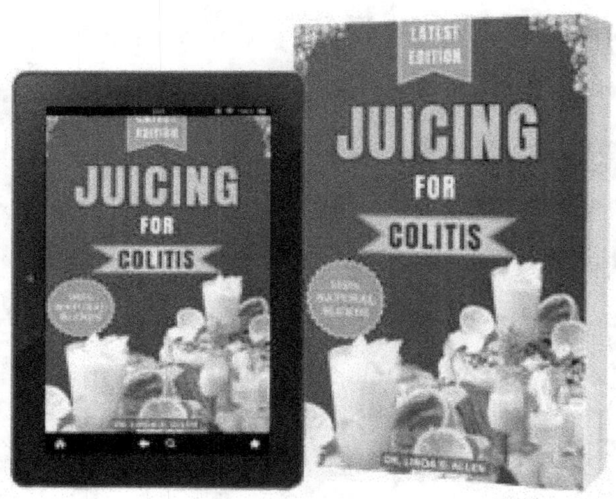

LATEST
EDITION
JUICING
FOR
COLITIS

INTRODUCTION

I Dr. Linda B. Allen, a seasoned expert in nutrition and dietetics, extend a warm and knowledgeable embrace to guide you through the transformative journey detailed in "Juicing for Colitis: 40 Essential and Easy-to-Make Nutrient-Rich Juice Blends for Crohn's, IBD, and Ulcerative Colitis Disease Management."

With years of experience dedicated to unraveling the intricacies of nutritional science and the human body's response to dietary interventions, I have witnessed firsthand the profound impact that targeted dietary measures can have on the management and alleviation of various health conditions. Specializing in nutrition and diet, my passion lies in empowering individuals to embrace a lifestyle that not only nourishes the body but also supports its inherent capacity to heal.

In this comprehensive guide, we delve into the realm of colitis, a condition that affects millions worldwide, exploring its nuances and unveiling a holistic approach to its management.

Colitis, a term often used to describe inflammation of the colon, encompasses a spectrum of disorders, including Crohn's disease, inflammatory bowel disease (IBD), and ulcerative colitis. Understanding the intricate interplay between nutrition and colitis is paramount, and this book serves as a beacon of knowledge, shedding light on effective dietary practices tailored for those navigating the challenges of colitis.

The journey begins with a profound exploration into the heart of colitis disease. What is colitis, and how does it manifest within the intricate landscape of the digestive system? We dissect the causes, unraveling the multifaceted origins of this condition that can be as complex and varied as the individuals it affects.

Armed with a profound understanding of colitis, we transition seamlessly into the heart of our guide - the tips and tricks of juicing for colitis. Drawing upon my extensive background in nutrition and dietetics, I unravel the intricacies of why juicing stands as a powerful ally in the management of colitis.

In the world of juicing, the right equipment acts as a trusted companion. As an experienced doctor in nutrition, I guide you through the labyrinth of juicing equipment, offering insights into the types, features, and recommendations tailored specifically for colitis-friendly juicing. It's not merely about extracting juice; it's about doing so in a manner that preserves the integrity of nutrients while catering to the sensitivities of a compromised digestive system.

Diving into the heart of juicing is an art that involves a thoughtful selection of ingredients. With my expertise as a nutrition and diet specialist, I meticulously outline nutrient-rich ingredients that not only support the nutritional needs of those grappling with colitis but also avoid triggering exacerbations.

Juicing is not merely about the act of creation; it extends to the art of preservation. Drawing from my extensive knowledge, I provide practical tips on how to store your precious creations, ensuring that each sip retains its nutritional potency. From the right containers to ideal storage conditions, this section ensures that your efforts in juicing are not just fruitful but sustainable in the long run.

The heart of the guide pulsates with life through 40 carefully curated juice blend recipes. Each recipe is a symphony of flavors, colors, and nutrients, meticulously crafted to not only tantalize the taste buds but to nourish the body and provide relief to those grappling with colitis. From soothing evening elixirs to Cherry Almond Protein Shake, this section transforms juicing into a delightful and therapeutic ritual.

Embark on this transformative odyssey with me as your guide, and together, let's unlock the potential of juicing for colitis, not just as a remedy but as a lifestyle that celebrates the profound connection between nutrition, well-being, and the body's innate capacity for healing.

PART 1

UNDERSTANDING COLITIS DISEASE

Colitis, an umbrella term referring to the inflammation of the colon, is a condition that impacts the digestive system, often leading to discomfort and disruptions in daily life. In this section, we aim to demystify colitis, offering you a clear understanding of the condition, its causes, signs and symptoms, and proactive measures to enhance prevention and management.

What is Colitis?

Colitis, simply put, is the inflammation of the colon, also known as the large intestine. This inflammation can arise from various factors, triggering a range of symptoms that affect the overall digestive process. Colitis isn't a singular ailment but rather a collective term encompassing conditions such as Crohn's disease, inflammatory bowel disease (IBD), and ulcerative colitis, each with its distinct characteristics and impact on the digestive system.

Causes of Colitis Disease

Understanding the causes of colitis is crucial in developing a targeted approach to its management. While the exact cause remains elusive and may vary among individuals, several factors contribute to the development of colitis. These include:

Immune System Dysfunction: Colitis is often linked to an abnormal immune response where the body's defense system mistakenly attacks the healthy cells in the colon.

Genetic Predisposition: There is evidence suggesting a genetic component to colitis. People who have an inflammatory bowel disease family history may be more susceptible.

Environmental Factors: External factors, such as certain infections or exposure to specific environmental elements, may trigger colitis in susceptible individuals.

Dietary Habits: While not a direct cause, certain dietary habits may exacerbate symptoms. High-fat diets, low fiber intake, and certain food sensitivities can contribute to inflammation.

Signs and Symptoms

Recognizing the signs and symptoms of colitis is pivotal for early intervention and effective management. Symptoms can vary in intensity and may include:

Abdominal Pain: Persistent discomfort or cramping in the abdominal region is a common symptom.

Diarrhea or Constipation: Fluctuations in bowel habits, ranging from diarrhea to constipation, may signal colitis.

Rectal Bleeding: Blood in the stool or during bowel movements is a significant red flag.

Weight Loss: Unexplained weight loss may occur due to nutrient malabsorption.

Fatigue: Chronic inflammation can lead to fatigue and a general sense of malaise.

Preventive Measures for Colitis

While colitis can be influenced by a combination of genetic and environmental factors, adopting preventive measures can significantly reduce the risk of its onset and alleviate symptoms. Consider the following proactive strategies:

Healthy Diet: Embrace a well-balanced diet rich in fiber, fruits, vegetables, and lean proteins. Avoid excessive consumption of processed foods and high-fat items.

Hydration: Maintain optimal hydration levels to support digestive functions and overall health.

Regular Exercise: Engage in regular physical activity to promote a healthy immune system and reduce inflammation.

Stress Management: Chronic stress can exacerbate colitis symptoms. Incorporate stress-reducing practices such as meditation, yoga, or deep-breathing exercises into your routine.

Regular Check-ups: Attend regular health check-ups, especially if you have a family history of inflammatory bowel diseases, to detect and address potential issues early.

PART 2

In this section, we'll explore practical tips and tricks for effective juicing, as well as Choosing the Right Juicing Equipment, Choosing the Juicing Ingredients, and How to Perfectly Store Your Juice.

Tips and Tricks of Juicing for Colitis

Start Slowly: If you're new to juicing, begin with small amounts and diluted blends. This allows your digestive system to adapt gradually to the influx of nutrients without overwhelming your gut.

Opt for Fresh Ingredients: Choose fresh, organic fruits and vegetables whenever possible. Fresh produce ensures maximum nutrient content and reduces the risk of additives that might trigger colitis symptoms.

Include Gut-Friendly Ingredients: Incorporate ingredients known for their gut-soothing properties. Aloe vera, ginger, and mint can provide a calming effect on the digestive system.

Experiment with Blends: Variety is key to a well-rounded nutritional intake. Experiment with different combinations of fruits and vegetables to discover blends that both please your palate and support your digestive health.

Remove Skin and Seeds: For certain fruits and vegetables, like apples and cucumbers, removing the skin and seeds can reduce fiber content and make the juice gentler on your digestive system.

Consider Nutrient Supplements: In consultation with your healthcare provider, consider adding nutrient supplements to your juice, especially if colitis has impacted nutrient absorption.

Choosing the Right Juicing Equipment

Centrifugal vs. Masticating Juicers: Centrifugal juicers are quicker but may generate heat, potentially impacting nutrient content. Masticating juicers operate at lower speeds, preserving more nutrients and minimizing heat production. Choose based on your preferences and health considerations.

Easy to Clean: Opt for juicers that are easy to disassemble and clean. Cleaning convenience ensures that juicing remains a sustainable and hassle-free part of your routine.

Juicing Speeds: Some juicers offer variable speeds, allowing you to juice soft and hard produce efficiently. Consider your preferred ingredients and select a juicer that accommodates your needs.

Pulp Extraction: If you prefer a smoother juice, choose a juicer with effective pulp extraction. However, some may enjoy the added fiber in their juice for its digestive benefits.

Choosing the Juicing Ingredients

Leafy Greens: Incorporate nutrient-dense leafy greens like kale, spinach, and Swiss chard. These greens are rich in vitamins and minerals while being gentle on the digestive system.

Low-Fiber Fruits: Opt for fruits low in insoluble fiber, such as bananas, melons, and cooked apples. These choices provide sweetness without overburdening the digestive tract.

Herbs for Flavor: Enhance the taste of your juice with digestive-friendly herbs like mint, cilantro, or basil. Not only do they add flavor, but they also offer additional health benefits.

Hydration Boosters: Include hydrating ingredients like cucumber and watermelon to boost your juice's liquid content, aiding in hydration and digestion.

How to Perfectly Store Your Juice

Use Airtight Containers: Store your juice in airtight containers to prevent oxidation and preserve freshness. Mason jars or glass bottles with tight-sealing lids work well.

Minimize Air Exposure: The less air your juice is exposed to, the better. Fill containers to the brim to minimize the surface area exposed to air.

Refrigerate Promptly: Refrigerate your juice immediately after preparation. Cold temperatures slow down the degradation of nutrients and inhibit the growth of harmful bacteria.

Consume Promptly: While freshly juiced is best, if you need to store your juice, aim to consume it within 24-48 hours to maximize its nutritional benefits.

By incorporating these tips and tricks into your juicing routine, you can make this therapeutic practice an enjoyable and effective part of your colitis management strategy.

PART 3

NOURISHING JUICE BLEND RECIPES

1. Soothing Green Elixir

Ingredients:

- 2 cups spinach leaves
- 1 cucumber (peeled if preferred)
- 1/2 cup fresh mint leaves
- 1 green apple (cored)
- 1 teaspoon fresh ginger (peeled)

Preparation:

- Wash all ingredients thoroughly.
- Run the spinach, cucumber, mint, apple, and ginger through the juicer.
- Stir well and pour over ice if desired.

Portion Size: One serving

Time:

- 10 minutes

Nutritional Information: Rich in vitamins A, C, and K, along with antioxidants and anti-inflammatory properties.

2. Citrus Burst Delight

Ingredients:

- 2 oranges (peeled)
- 1 grapefruit (peeled)
- 1 lemon (peeled)
- 1 tablespoon fresh turmeric (peeled)

Preparation:

1. Peel the oranges, grapefruit, lemon, and turmeric.
2. Juice the peeled fruits and turmeric.
3. Mix well and serve chilled.

Portion Size: One serving

Time: 10 minutes

Nutritional Information: Packed with immune-boosting vitamin C, anti-inflammatory compounds, and digestive enzymes.

3. Carrot-Ginger Zest

Ingredients:

- 4 large carrots (peeled)
- 1 apple (cored)
- 1 tablespoon fresh ginger (peeled)

Preparation:

1. Peel and chop the carrots, core the apple, and peel the ginger.
2. Juice the carrots, apple, and ginger.
3. Stir well and enjoy immediately.

Portion Size: One serving

Time: 10 minutes

Nutritional Information: High in beta-carotene, vitamin A, and anti-inflammatory properties.

4. Pineapple-Kale Harmony

Ingredients:

- 1 cup fresh pineapple chunks
- 2 cups kale leaves (stems removed)
- 1 cucumber (peeled)
- 1 lime (peeled)

Preparation:

1. Cut the pineapple into chunks, peel the cucumber, and remove the stems from the kale.
2. Juice the pineapple, kale, cucumber, and lime.
3. Mix well and serve over ice if desired.

Portion Size: One serving

Time: 10 minutes

Nutritional Information: Packed with vitamin C, bromelain (anti-inflammatory enzyme), and fiber.

5. Berry Bliss Infusion

Ingredients:

- 1 cup mixed berries (blueberries, raspberries, strawberries)
- 1 pear (cored)
- 1/2 cup fresh basil leaves

Preparation:

1. Wash the berries and basil, and core the pear.
2. Juice the mixed berries, pear, and basil.
3. Stir well and serve chilled.

Portion Size: One serving

Time: 10 minutes

Nutritional Information: Rich in antioxidants, vitamins, and anti-inflammatory properties.

6. Healing Minty Pineapple Twist

Ingredients:

- 1 cup pineapple chunks
- 1 cucumber (peeled)
- 1/2 cup fresh mint leaves
- 1 teaspoon chia seeds (optional)

Preparation:

1. Peel the cucumber and cut it into chunks.
2. Juice the pineapple, cucumber, and mint.
3. Stir in chia seeds if desired and let it sit for a few minutes to absorb liquid.
4. Serve over ice.

Portion Size: One serving

Time: 10 minutes

Nutritional Information: Rich in bromelain (anti-inflammatory enzyme), mint for digestive comfort, and hydrating cucumber.

7. Blueberry-Ginger Infusion

Ingredients:

- 1 cup blueberries
- 1 apple (cored)
- 1 tablespoon fresh ginger (peeled)
- 1 teaspoon flaxseeds (optional)

Preparation:

1. Core the apple and peel the ginger.
2. Juice the blueberries, apple, and ginger.
3. Stir in flaxseeds if desired.
4. Serve immediately.

Portion Size: One serving

Time: 10 minutes

Nutritional Information: High in antioxidants from blueberries, anti-inflammatory ginger, and optional flaxseeds for added omega-3s.

8. Cucumber-Celery Refresher

Ingredients:

- 2 cucumbers (peeled)
- 4 celery stalks
- 1/2 lemon (peeled)
- 1 tablespoon fresh parsley

Preparation:

1. Peel the cucumbers and lemon, and chop them into manageable pieces.
2. Juice the cucumbers, celery, lemon, and parsley.
3. Stir well and pour over ice if desired.

Portion Size: One serving

Time: 10 minutes

Nutritional Information: Hydrating cucumber, celery for digestive support, and lemon for a burst of vitamin C.

9. Papaya-Coconut Bliss

Ingredients:

- 1 cup ripe papaya chunks
- 1/2 cup coconut water
- 1/2 cup pineapple chunks
- 1 tablespoon fresh lime juice

Preparation:

1. Peel and seed the papaya, cut it into chunks.
2. Juice the papaya, coconut water, pineapple, and lime.
3. Stir well and serve chilled.

Portion Size: One serving

Time: 10 minutes

Nutritional Information: Papaya for digestive enzymes, coconut water for hydration, and pineapple for bromelain.

10. Spinach-Berry Delight

Ingredients:

- 2 cups fresh spinach leaves
- One cup of mixed berries, including raspberries, blueberries, and strawberries.
- 1 apple (cored)
- 1/2 lemon (peeled)

Preparation:

1. Core the apple and peel the lemon.
2. Juice the spinach, mixed berries, apple, and lemon.
3. Stir well and serve over ice if desired.

Portion Size: One serving

Time: 10 minutes

Nutritional Information: Spinach for iron and vitamins, mixed berries for antioxidants, and apple for natural sweetness.

11. Tropical Turmeric Elixir

Ingredients:

- 1 cup pineapple chunks
- 1 orange (peeled)
- 1 teaspoon fresh turmeric (peeled)
- 1/2 teaspoon coconut oil

Preparation:

1. Peel the orange and turmeric.
2. Juice the pineapple, orange, and turmeric.
3. Add coconut oil and blend until smooth.
4. Serve immediately.

Portion Size: One serving

Time: 10 minutes

Nutritional Information: Pineapple for bromelain, orange for vitamin C, turmeric for anti-inflammatory properties, and coconut oil for healthy fats.

12. Kale-Apple Zinger

Ingredients:

- 2 cups kale leaves (stems removed)
- 2 apples (cored)
- 1/2 lemon (peeled)
- 1-inch fresh ginger (peeled)

Preparation:

1. Core the apples, peel the lemon, and remove the stems from kale.
2. Juice the kale, apples, lemon, and ginger.
3. Stir well and serve over ice if desired.

Portion Size: One serving

Time: 10 minutes

Nutritional Information: Kale for vitamins A and K, apples for natural sweetness, lemon for vitamin C, and ginger for digestive support.

13. Minty Melon Soother

Ingredients:

- 2 cups watermelon chunks
- 1 cucumber (peeled)
- 1/2 cup fresh mint leaves
- 1 lime (peeled)

Preparation:

1. Peel the cucumber and lime.
2. Juice the watermelon, cucumber, mint, and lime.
3. Stir well and serve chilled.

Portion Size: One serving

Time: 10 minutes

Nutritional Information: Hydrating watermelon, cucumber for digestive comfort, mint for flavor, and lime for a burst of vitamin C.

14. Beet-Berry Vitalizer

Ingredients:

- 1 medium beet (peeled)
- 1 cup mixed berries (blueberries, raspberries, strawberries)
- 1 apple (cored)
- 1/2 lemon (peeled)

Preparation:

1. Peel the beet, core the apple, and peel the lemon.
2. Juice the beet, mixed berries, apple, and lemon.
3. Stir well and serve immediately.

Portion Size: One serving

Time: 10 minutes

Nutritional Information: Beets for folate and antioxidants, mixed berries for vitamins, apple for natural sweetness, and lemon for vitamin C.

15. Carrot-Orange Elegance

Ingredients:

- 4 large carrots (peeled)
- 2 oranges (peeled)
- 1-inch fresh ginger (peeled)

Preparation:

1. Peel the carrots, oranges, and ginger.
2. Juice the carrots, oranges, and ginger.
3. Stir well and serve over ice if desired.

Portion Size: One serving

Time: 10 minutes

Nutritional Information: Carrots for beta-carotene, oranges for vitamin C, and ginger for anti-inflammatory properties.

16. Berry Basil Bliss

Ingredients:

- 1 cup mixed berries (blueberries, raspberries, strawberries)
- 1 pear (cored)
- 1/2 cup fresh basil leaves
- 1 tablespoon chia seeds

Preparation:

1. Wash the berries and basil, and core the pear.
2. Juice the mixed berries, pear, and basil.
3. Stir in chia seeds and let it sit for a few minutes.
4. Serve chilled.

Portion Size: One serving

Time: 10 minutes

Nutritional Information: Berries for antioxidants, pear for fiber, basil for flavor, and chia seeds for omega-3s.

17. Spinach-Pineapple Refresher

Ingredients:

- 2 cups fresh spinach leaves
- 1 cup pineapple chunks
- 1 cucumber (peeled)
- 1/2 lime (peeled)

Preparation:

1. Peel the cucumber and lime.
2. Juice the spinach, pineapple, cucumber, and lime.
3. Stir well and serve over ice if desired.

Portion Size: One serving

Time: 10 minutes

Nutritional Information: Spinach for vitamins and minerals, pineapple for bromelain, cucumber for hydration, and lime for vitamin C.

18. Cooling Cabbage Citrus

Ingredients:

- 1 cup green cabbage
- 2 oranges (peeled)
- 1 apple (cored)
- 1/2 lemon (peeled)

Preparation:

1. Core the apple, peel the oranges and lemon, and chop the cabbage.
2. Juice the cabbage, oranges, apple, and lemon.
3. Stir well and serve chilled.

Portion Size: One serving

Time: 10 minutes

Nutritional Information: Cabbage for anti-inflammatory compounds, oranges for vitamin C, apple for natural sweetness, and lemon for flavor.

19. Avocado-Grapefruit Elegance

Ingredients:

- 1 avocado (peeled and pitted)
- 1 grapefruit (peeled)
- 1 cucumber (peeled)
- 1 tablespoon fresh mint leaves

Preparation:

1. Peel the avocado, grapefruit, and cucumber.
2. Juice the avocado, grapefruit, cucumber, and mint.
3. Blend until smooth.
4. Serve immediately.

Portion Size: One serving

Time: 10 minutes

Nutritional Information: Avocado for healthy fats, grapefruit for antioxidants, cucumber for hydration, and mint for digestive comfort.

20. Tomato-Basil Infusion

Ingredients:

- 2 large tomatoes
- 1 cucumber (peeled)
- 1/2 cup fresh basil leaves
- 1/2 lemon (peeled)

Preparation:

1. Peel the cucumber and lemon.
2. Juice the tomatoes, cucumber, basil, and lemon.
3. Stir well and serve over ice if desired.

Portion Size: One serving

Time: 10 minutes

Nutritional Information: Tomatoes for lycopene, cucumber for hydration, basil for flavor, and lemon for vitamin C.

1. Blueberry Banana Bliss

Ingredients:

- 1 cup blueberries
- 1 banana
- 1/2 cup Greek yogurt
- 1 tablespoon chia seeds

Preparation:

1. Blend blueberries, banana, Greek yogurt, and chia seeds until smooth.
2. Serve immediately.

Portion Size: One serving

Time: 5 minutes

Nutritional Information: Blueberries for antioxidants, banana for potassium, Greek yogurt for probiotics, and chia seeds for omega-3s.

2. Spinach Mango Delight

Ingredients:

- 2 cups fresh spinach leaves
- 1 cup mango chunks
- 1/2 cucumber (peeled)
- 1/2 cup coconut water

Preparation:

1. Blend spinach, mango, cucumber, and coconut water until smooth.
2. Serve over ice if desired.

Portion Size: One serving

Time: 5 minutes

Nutritional Information: Spinach for vitamins and minerals, mango for vitamin C, cucumber for hydration, and coconut water for electrolytes.

3. Kiwi Pineapple Refresher

Ingredients:

- 2 kiwis (peeled)
- 1 cup pineapple chunks
- 1/2 cup Greek yogurt
- 1 tablespoon honey (optional)

Preparation:

1. Blend kiwis, pineapple, Greek yogurt, and honey until smooth.
2. Serve chilled.

Portion Size: One serving

Time: 5 minutes

Nutritional Information: Kiwi for vitamin C, pineapple for bromelain, Greek yogurt for probiotics, and honey for sweetness.

4. Papaya Coconut Smoothie Bowl

Ingredients:

- 1 cup ripe papaya chunks
- 1/2 cup coconut milk
- 1/4 cup granola
- 1 tablespoon shredded coconut

Preparation:

1. Blend papaya and coconut milk until smooth.
2. Pour into a bowl and top with granola and shredded coconut.

Portion Size: One serving

Time: 5 minutes

Nutritional Information: Papaya for digestive enzymes, coconut milk for healthy fats, granola for fiber, and shredded coconut for flavor.

5. Carrot Apple Ginger Elixir

Ingredients:

- 3 medium carrots (peeled)
- 2 apples (cored)
- 1 tablespoon fresh ginger (peeled)
- 1/2 lemon (peeled)

Preparation:

1. Blend carrots, apples, ginger, and lemon until smooth.
2. Serve over ice if desired.

Portion Size: One serving

Time: 5 minutes

Nutritional Information: Carrots for beta-carotene, apples for natural sweetness, ginger for anti-inflammatory properties, and lemon for vitamin C.

6. Pineapple Basil Citrus Splash

Ingredients:

- 1 cup pineapple chunks
- 1 orange (peeled)
- 1/2 lemon (peeled)
- 1/4 cup fresh basil leaves

Preparation:

1. Blend pineapple, orange, lemon, and basil until smooth.
2. Serve chilled.

Portion Size: One serving

Time: 5 minutes

Nutritional Information: Pineapple for bromelain, orange for vitamin C, lemon for flavor, and basil for digestive comfort.

7. Banana Almond Protein Boost

Ingredients:

- 2 bananas
- 1/2 cup almond butter
- 1 cup almond milk
- 1 tablespoon flaxseeds

Preparation:

1. Blend bananas, almond butter, almond milk, and flaxseeds until smooth.
2. Serve immediately.

Portion Size: One serving

Time: 5 minutes

Nutritional Information: Bananas for potassium, almond butter for healthy fats, almond milk for calcium, and flaxseeds for omega-3s.

8. Berry Oatmeal Power Smoothie

Ingredients:

- One cup of mixed berries, including raspberries, blueberries, and strawberries.
- 1/2 cup rolled oats
- 1/2 cup Greek yogurt
- 1 tablespoon honey (optional)

Preparation:

1. Blend mixed berries, rolled oats, Greek yogurt, and honey until smooth.
2. Serve chilled.

Portion Size: One serving

Time: 5 minutes

Nutritional Information: Berries for antioxidants, oats for fiber, Greek yogurt for probiotics, and honey for sweetness.

9. Avocado Lime Green Goodness

Ingredients:

- 1/2 avocado (peeled and pitted)
- 1 cup kale leaves (stems removed)
- 1/2 cucumber (peeled)
- 1/2 lime (peeled)

Preparation:

1. Blend avocado, kale, cucumber, and lime until smooth.
2. Serve over ice if desired.

Portion Size: One serving

Time: 5 minutes

Nutritional Information: Avocado for healthy fats, kale for vitamins, cucumber for hydration, and lime for vitamin C.

10. Melon Mint Hydrating Cooler

Ingredients:

- Two cups of chunky melon (honeydew, or cantaloupe)
- 1/2 cup coconut water
- 1/4 cup fresh mint leaves
- 1 tablespoon chia seeds

Preparation:

1. Blend melon, coconut water, mint, and chia seeds until smooth.
2. Serve chilled.

Portion Size: One serving

Time: 5 minutes

Nutritional Information: Melon for hydration, coconut water for electrolytes, mint for flavor, and chia seeds for omega-3s.

11. Green Tea Berry Boost

Ingredients:

- 1 cup mixed berries (blueberries, raspberries, strawberries)
- 1/2 cup brewed green tea (cooled)
- 1/2 banana
- 1 tablespoon chia seeds

Preparation:

1. Blend mixed berries, green tea, banana, and chia seeds until smooth.
2. Serve chilled.

Portion Size: One serving

Time: 5 minutes

Nutritional Information: Berries for antioxidants, green tea for anti-inflammatory compounds, banana for potassium, and chia seeds for omega-3s.

12. Almond Spinach Protein Shake

Ingredients:

- 2 cups fresh spinach leaves
- 1/2 cup almond milk
- 1/2 cup Greek yogurt
- 1 tablespoon almond butter

Preparation:

1. Blend spinach, almond milk, Greek yogurt, and almond butter until smooth.
2. Serve over ice if desired.

Portion Size: One serving

Time: 5 minutes

Nutritional Information: Spinach for vitamins and minerals, almond milk for calcium, Greek yogurt for probiotics, and almond butter for healthy fats.

13. Turmeric Mango Lassi

Ingredients:

- 1 cup mango chunks
- 1/2 cup plain yogurt
- 1/2 teaspoon fresh turmeric (peeled)
- 1 tablespoon honey (optional)

Preparation:

1. Blend mango, yogurt, turmeric, and honey until smooth.
2. Serve chilled.

Portion Size: One serving

Time: 5 minutes

Nutritional Information: Mango for vitamin C, yogurt for probiotics, turmeric for anti-inflammatory properties, and honey for sweetness.

14. Raspberry Coconut Bliss

Ingredients:

- 1 cup raspberries
- 1/2 cup coconut milk
- 1/2 banana
- 1 tablespoon shredded coconut

Preparation:

1. Blend raspberries, coconut milk, banana, and shredded coconut until smooth.
2. Serve immediately.

Portion Size: One serving

Time: 5 minutes

Nutritional Information: Raspberries for antioxidants, coconut milk for healthy fats, banana for potassium, and shredded coconut for flavor.

15. Peach Mint Relaxation Smoothie

Ingredients:

- 2 peaches (peeled and pitted)
- 1/2 cup fresh mint leaves
- 1/2 cucumber (peeled)
- 1/2 lemon (peeled)

Preparation:

1. Blend peaches, mint, cucumber, and lemon until smooth.
2. Serve over ice if desired.

Portion Size: One serving

Time: 5 minutes

Nutritional Information: Peaches for vitamins A and C, mint for digestive comfort, cucumber for hydration, and lemon for vitamin C.

16. Berry Avocado Power Shake

Ingredients:

- One cup of mixed berries, comprising blueberries, strawberries, and raspberries.
- 1/2 avocado (peeled and pitted)
- 1/2 cup almond milk
- 1 tablespoon flaxseeds

Preparation:

1. Blend mixed berries, avocado, almond milk, and flaxseeds until smooth.
2. Serve chilled.

Portion Size: One serving

Time: 5 minutes

Nutritional Information: Berries for antioxidants, avocado for healthy fats, almond milk for calcium, and flaxseeds for omega-3s.

17. Orange Carrot Ginger Zinger

Ingredients:

- 2 oranges (peeled)
- 4 large carrots (peeled)
- 1 tablespoon fresh ginger (peeled)
- 1 tablespoon honey (optional)

Preparation:

1. Blend oranges, carrots, ginger, and honey until smooth.
2. Serve over ice if desired.

Portion Size: One serving

Time: 5 minutes

Nutritional Information: Oranges for vitamin C, carrots for beta-carotene, ginger for anti-inflammatory properties, and honey for sweetness.

18. Blueberry Coconut Protein Punch

Ingredients:

- 1 cup blueberries
- 1/2 cup coconut water
- 1/2 cup Greek yogurt
- 1 tablespoon chia seeds

Preparation:

1. Blend blueberries, coconut water, Greek yogurt, and chia seeds until smooth.
2. Serve chilled.

Portion Size: One serving

Time: 5 minutes

Nutritional Information: Blueberries for antioxidants, coconut water for electrolytes, Greek yogurt for probiotics, and chia seeds for omega-3s.

19. Cucumber Pineapple Hydration Cooler

Ingredients:

- 1/2 cucumber (peeled)
- 1 cup pineapple chunks
- 1/2 cup coconut water
- 1 tablespoon fresh mint leaves

Preparation:

- Blend cucumber, pineapple, coconut water, and mint until smooth.
- Serve over ice if desired.

Portion Size: One serving

Time: 5 minutes

Nutritional Information: Cucumber for hydration, pineapple for bromelain, coconut water for electrolytes, and mint for digestive comfort.

20. Cherry Almond Protein Shake

Ingredients:

- 1 cup cherries (pitted)
- 1/2 cup almond milk
- 1/2 cup Greek yogurt
- 1 tablespoon almond butter

Preparation:

1. Blend cherries, almond milk, Greek yogurt, and almond butter until smooth.
2. Serve immediately.

Portion Size: One serving

Time: 5 minutes

Nutritional Information: Cherries for antioxidants, almond milk for calcium, Greek yogurt for probiotics, and almond butter for healthy fats.

CONCLUSION

Throughout the book, we delved into the fundamentals of understanding colitis, exploring its nature, causes, signs, symptoms, and preventive measures. By gaining a deeper understanding of the disease, you been equipped with the knowledge necessary to make informed choices regarding their dietary habits and overall well-being.

The book then shifted focus to the art and science of juicing for colitis, presenting valuable tips and tricks. From selecting the right juicing equipment to choosing ingredients that are gentle on the digestive system, the guidance provided aims to empower readers to integrate juicing into their daily routine effectively. Emphasis has been placed on the significance of proper storage to retain the nutritional integrity of the juices.

The heart of the book lies in the 40 nourishing juice blend and smoothie recipes, meticulously crafted to not only cater to the nutritional needs of individuals with colitis but also to tantalize the taste buds.

Each recipe is a fusion of flavors, colors, and health benefits, carefully curated to support digestion, reduce inflammation, and promote overall well-being. From soothing evening elixirs to Cherry Almond Protein Shake, these recipes offer a diverse array of options for individuals to enjoy as they embark on their colitis management journey.

I encourage you to view this book as a companion on your path to colitis recovery. It is my sincere hope that the information and recipes provided serve as a source of inspiration, fostering a positive relationship with nutrition and wellness. Remember, individual responses to dietary changes may vary, and it is crucial to consult with healthcare professionals for personalized advice.

In closing, may this book stand as a beacon of support for those navigating the challenges of colitis, offering not only nourishment for the body but also a sense of empowerment and hope for a healthier tomorrow.

Here's to your health and vitality as you embark on this transformative journey.

9 798877 129672